The Number One Secret To Permanent Weight Loss

By Arthur Guess

Ch.1 Journey To The Secret

Hello, I have written this book with the hope of helping others who have suffered as I have suffered for
years with overweight and overeating and I have purposefully made it a short read so that length of time in reading it will not be an excuse not to read it. I don't think a book like this need to be a war and peace read that take you forever to get through if you finish it at all. Well it all started for me as a child I would sometimes overeat to the point of getting sick and throwing up. I would only do this a

few times a year so I don't consider that I was or am bulimic but I certainly had the potential to end up that way. I can remember going to a local church and when they had VBS the last night of it would be games and FOOD! I would stuff myself on hot dogs and chips and then go throw up so I could eat some more. I was raised dirt poor and we didn't always have a good availability of food and if it weren't for food stamps back then we probably all would have starved. My father raised six of us on less than 15,000 a year so there were a lot of times when there wasn't much food. I can remember going to friends' house and playing with them and then hoping to be invited to stay for dinner. My mother bless her heart, on top of not having a lot of food she wasn't what I would call a world class chef either. Sometimes she would burn the food etc. but she did the best she could.

I enter into my teen years and wasn't what you would call really fat but I was of a stocky build and I absolutely loved school food. For me that was the highlight of each day was lunch because usually lunch was breakfast and lunch for me as my mother never fixed us breakfast before school and sometimes the school provided breakfast but not always.

I began working full time at the age of 16 at Kentucky Fried Chicken and moved out of my parents house to live with and split the rent with my brother. I knew as poor as I was being raised that I could fare better and have a better standard of living on my own with my brother so that is what I did and I loved it. He treated me like and adult and I pretty much came and went as I pleased and I felt that I was very responsible for a teenager and was mature enough to handle it and so I did.

It was about this time that I met my future wife to be and we started dating-that's when the weight started going up. Oh my word can her mama cook! I had never eaten such delicious food in my life except for my grandmother who I didn't get to see very often. I put on about 20 pounds after a month of dating and then another 20 after quitting smoking and that will be for another book of how I quit smoking . So now I was up to 220 pounds and so began my place in hell with all the other sufferers of overeating and dieting and add infinitum. I tried eating less and drinking more and exercising only to fail over and over again. I would have some success but then somehow manage to put the weight back on and even more.

I tried Weight Watchers and Atkins and Sugar Busters and most of them all starved me to death or made me very unhappy because I could not eat the things I love. I will that I had the most success with a low carb approach modified for me to include the things I love. If you love ice cream and it is not part of you "diet" you will not stay on that diet. Everyone is on a diet, all a diet means is the particular things that you personally choose or don't choose to eat.

I was on a quest to find the best type of eating for my body type. Everyone has a different body type and different metabolism which is the rate at which your body burns food. If you are someone who has a very slow metabolism then the things most diets recommend you to eat will actually make you gain weight. You can get just as fat off of fruits and vegetables as you can from candy and doughnuts. Please hear me on this, THERE IS NO SUCH THING AS BAD FOOD.Certain foods are better for your health than others but Food is food and to say this is bad or don't ever eat this sets you up for what I call Eve's Syndrome-that which you can't have or is taboo is do or die to get it -what you can't have you want the most so some things will be right for your unique body and some things will be like poison to your body. You must be your own scientist and researcher and start doing experiments with food. Eat certain things for breakfast and see how you feel then try other things and see how long it lasts you and absolutely weigh yourself every day in the morning before eating or drinking anything. If you work nights then weigh yourself whenever you first get up regardless if it is night of day and if you have a gain think of what you ate the day before and make note of it. If you have trouble remembering it is a great idea to keep a notebook handy or just some scrap paper that you keep up with what your eating and write it down. You will begin to see what foods and amounts make you gain and what foods and amounts make you lose.

Ch.2 Spirituality

You may think it very strange that I would include a chapter on spiritual matters but I feel it something that must not be overlooked. I personally believe we are spiritual beings temporarily housed in physical bodies and so it is of utmost importance on your journey to permanent weight loss to make sure you have matters that are spiritual squared away between you and your God. If you don't believe in God I totally respect that and it is every persons' individual right to choose to believe as they wish. I personally believe in Jesus Christ and that he has been a great help to me in my life. If you believe in Buddha or whomever is your God you be at peace within yourself about it and if you are not do the research and try out all the religions and learn about them and go with what you feel you should.

I know the main difference between Christianity and all other world religions is that they all are a works based religion to get to Heaven, Nirvana or whatever. Christianity is somewhat different in that it teaches you could never be good enough or work hard enough to measure up to God's Standard so he met the standard for you through his son Jesus by dying on the cross for your sins. None of us and I mean none of us are sinless. You find the most holy and righteous person on the Earth today and if you were allowed to examine their life close enough you will find sin. If any of us could have ever been sinless there would not have been a need for Christ to die on the cross for us. So for what I believe it is only through faith in Christ that saves us from our sinful condition. Ok with that having been said again this is my personal belief, if you disagree that is fine we can agree to disagree and go on in love and not worry about it.

The reason I wanted to focus on this some is that if you are not in harmony and at peace with your God, the universe and people around you including family it will be very difficult to attain permanent weight loss because if your spirit is out of balance it will show up in you body in excess weight or some other malady possible even worse that just being overweight. If you are not sure how to go about this I highly recommend you look into Overeaters Anonymous or similar support group with an emphasis on spirituality.

Ch. 3 The Secret

This is the chapter that gets down to why you probably bought this booklet to begin with and that is the secret to permanent weight loss. What is it, what's it look like, smell like, taste like, and how do I get it. Well the secret is simple, are you ready, here it is! The secret is YOU! That's right the secret to permanent weight loss lies within you and your desire to accomplish it. You have to desire this like you have never desired anything in your life and it will happen once you have the desire. The reason I believe this is that it is only with the desire that the groundwork and footwork will occur that will bring you to what is the best way of eating for your particular body type and what kind of exercise you may or may not incorporate into your new lifestyle. Please understand this also-you do not have to exercise to lose weight! Am I saying this is the best way to go about it, absolutely not, you should exercise and it is best for you if you do adopt a regular exercise program but let's face it, many of us will not and if that is what it takes then many will never lose the excess pounds. That is why I am here to tell you that you don't have to exercise to lose the weight. To lose weight it is as simple as EATING LESS THAN YOUR BODY NEEDS WILL CAUSE WEIGHT LOSS AND EATING MORE THAN YOU BODY NEEDS WILL ADD WEIGHT. I don't care what the foods are that you eat it comes down to the amounts. You can eat candy every day and lose weight. I did it on my modified low carb approach, I would eat 4 to 5 miniature peanut butter cups almost everyday and I lost 50 pounds. I originally got up to 285 pounds a few years ago and I was full blown diabetic with hemoglobin of 8.0 and I had high blood pressure and I started taking pills for blood pressure and diabetes and I figured if I wanted to be around to see my kids grow up I had better start doing something and that is when I really began to dig and research and find what was going to be the "secret" for me to lose weight and keep it off. I lost 50 pounds eating candy every day and I did not exercise once and just after losing 20 pounds the high blood pressure and diabetes literally went away! That's when I knew I was onto to something incredible! I am not saying this is the way to do it but it is the way I did it. The thing is in the amounts. If your body uses let's say 200 carbs a day to maintain a weight of 200 pounds and you eat 400 carbs a day you will be weighing in at 400 pounds before too long. Watch the amount you eat, if you normally eat a whole bag of chips, eat a half bag of chips and stop. If you eat 3 sandwiches for lunch, eat only two. Little cutbacks here and there will lower you total intake of carbs for the day and you will lose weight. The reason I say go by your carbs instead of calories is because it much easier to do math in your head when your talking about a couple of hundred or less, with calories you into the thousands and trying to keep track of it. Another thing you can do if you know you want to or are going to be eating a meal with lots of carbs all you have to do is eat extremely low carb for breakfast that day then eat pizza or whatever is high carb for lunch and then back to extremely low carb for dinner and your total carbs for the day will still be within the range you need them to be and you will not gain a pound. The only thing you have to be careful of with this is if the high carb food is a type that spikes your blood sugar so high that you starve to death later and overeat but this will be found out as you become your own nutritionist and experiment with different foods and see how they affect you. Also if you find yourself much like alcoholic is to alcohol and if food is like that to you then I cannot stress it enough and I cannot recommend it highly enough and that is to get involved with an Overeaters Anonymous or similar support group because there is hope for you no matter big you may be or how addicted to food you may be you can recover but remember, what is the secret? The secret is you and your desire for better health and doing anything it takes to achieve it even if that means humbling yourself and going to an OA meeting regularly. Just remember what other people think of you is basically not any of your business and just think how little time you actually spend thinking about others, that how much time they spend thinking about you. Most of us are wrapped up in our own little lives doing out thing so you do your thing and don't worry about what others will think. To give you an example on different foods and how they can affect you   I can eat a huge meal of breadsticks with cheese and dipping sauce and literally gain a couple of pounds overnight. Or I can eat a heavy meal rich in protein and low in carbs and not gain at all and even lose weight that way. But I still like and the breadsticks too, the difference is making room for things you love and not worrying about each meal. You only need to keep track of your carb intake. If you are extremely obese and your carb intake is around 400 to 500 or more do not expect to immediately get down to eating only 200 carbs a day. Your goal should be to get down to 400 carbs a day if you are eating 500 and if your eating 400 your goal should be to get down to 300. You must drop your carb intake gradually over a period of time so as not to put your mind and body in shock because of such a sudden change. Once you begin to lose weight you will be able to find what the ideal carb intake per day is for you particular body type. My metabolism is on the slow side so I can't go very high in carbs without seeing an immediate weight gain. It is also recommended that you not lose more than a couple of pounds a week is the safest way so if you are 200 pounds overweight if will take you a little over two years to lose that weight at the 2 pound a week loss. Don't be discouraged by this because most people will find they lose weight faster than that just don't be trying to starve yourself. Remember your goal is permanent weight loss and you don't get there by starving yourself, you get there by enjoying all foods in moderation.

I could go on into great detail about what all these different foods do in your body and explain all the other things with blood sugar and insulin etc etc. but that is where you come in and your DESIRE to achieve permanent weight loss. This is where you ignore everything everyone has told you about weight loss including me and you begin your quest for the key to it for you because your permanent "diet" will not like mine or anyone's else's. It will be yours and yours alone. You might like pigs' feet for all I know and that is fine just remember to include everything and I mean everything you love and do it in a responsible and moderate manner. Research as I did and each book and article you read about this only adds to your knowledge and educate yourself to reaching your ideal weight. Don't be afraid of reading books you have heard bad things about. Read it for yourself and use what you agree with and ignore those things you don't agree with. Once you reach your goal that is just part of the picture the rest of the picture is getting there on your terms and the way that fits you best so you don't have a crummy restrictive diet to go on or off of but you will have created your own way and your own 'diet for life' that includes everything you love in moderation as God intended.

The following pages are for 31 days for journal keeping to help you get started on your way to permanent weight loss!

Day One

For the next three days do not cut back at all on your eating. Just record what you eat here in this and figure where you are on your total carbohydrate intake on average for three day and then you will know what your goal carb total intake for each day should look like. Also it is best to try and just cut out snacking altogether unless you feel you are very disciplined and can do so without going over your carb total. I personally like to save my carb amout for a really awesome meal instead of wasting it on little things although I do like to snack occasionally on just about anything that is really low carb.

Breakfast

_____
_____
_____
_____
_____
_____
_____

_____

Lunch

_____
_____
_____
_____
_____
_____
_____

_____

Supper

_____
_____
_____
_____
_____
_____
_____

_____

Total Carb Intake

_____

Day Two

Remember to just record your
carbs to the right of the page so it
will
Easier to tally up.

Breakfast

_____
_____
_____
_____
_____
_____
_____
_____
_____

Lunch

_____
_____
_____
_____
_____
_____
_____
_____

_____

Supper

_____
_____
_____
_____
_____
_____
_____
_____

_____

Total Carbs

_____

Day Three

At the end of today or tomorrow morning total your carbs and come up with an average for the past three days and then decide your total goal for the next day.

Breakfast

_____

_____

_____

_____

_____

_____

_____

_____

_____

Lunch

_____

_____

_____

_____

_____

_____

_____

_____

_____

Supper

_____

_____

_____

_____

_____

_____

_____

_____

_____

Total Carbs

_____

Total Three Day Average of Carbs

_____-

Day Four

Now your ready this is the big day
to start eating less. Remember the
key is to slowly reduce over a long
period of time and you fall off the
wagon-who cares, big deal! Just
never ever never never never give
up, NEVER GIVE UP   and
NEVER GIVE UP keep at it and
you will have permanent weight
loss.

Breakfast

_____

_____

_____

_____

_____

_____

_____

_____

_____

Lunch

_____

_____

_____

_____

_____

_____

_____

_____

_____

Supper

_____

_____

_____

_____

_____

_____

_____

_____

_____

Total Carbs

_____

Day Five
Remember each brand new day is
brand new day to start again if you
didn't do so well yesterday but

think of this way of you normally
eat a whole bag of potatoe chips
and you only eat ¾ of a bag that is
A HUGE SUCCESS because you
normally ate the whole bag so
whatever small amout you are able
to change the amount is A STEP
IN THE RIGHT DIRECTION and
enough steps in the right direction
and suddenly you'll be at your
destination!

Breakfast

_____
_____
_____
_____
_____
_____
_____
_____
_____

Lunch

_____

_____

_____

_____

_____

_____

_____

_____

_____

Supper

_____

_____

_____

_____

_____

_____

_____

_____

_____

Total Carbs

_____

Day Six

Just keep at it Rome wasn't built in
day and neither was your big ole
butt!
So just plan your work and work
your plan.

Breakfast

_____
_____
_____
_____
_____
_____
_____
_____
_____

Lunch

_____

_____

_____

_____

_____

_____

_____

_____

Supper

_____

_____

_____

_____

_____

_____

Total Carbs

_____

Feel free to use extra space on the pages to to record you thoughts, what foods you ate and how they affected you good or bad and what foods put you completely out of control if any and what you are going to do about that. This is the only situation where I would reccomend totally not eating something ever is if your one bite of it puts you out of control, this is the only time you may have to give something up altogether and if you feel all food of any kind puts you out of control you will really need to seek professional help in additon to a support group.But I believe most can retrain their self to enjoy moderate amounts of anything.

Day Seven

Breakfast

_____

_____

_____

_____

_____

_____

_____

_____

Lunch

_____

_____

_____

_____

_____

_____

_____

_____

Supper

_____

_____

_____

_____

_____

_____

_____

_____

_____

Total Carbs

_____

Day Eight

If you are not familiar with counting carbs look on the nutrition label and subtract the fiber from the amount of carbohydrate for the most accurate count.

Breakfast

_____

_____

_____

_____

_____

_____

_____

_____

_____

Lunch

_____

_____

_____

_____

_____

_____

_____

_____

_____

Supper

_____

_____

_____

_____

_____

_____

_____

_____

_____

Total Carbs

_____

Day Nine

Breakfast

_____

_____

_____

_____

_____

_____

_____

_____

_____

Lunch

_____

_____

_____

_____

_____

_____

_____

_____

_____

Supper

_____

_____

_____

_____

_____

_____

_____

_____

_____

Total Carbs

_____

Day Ten

You should be getting the hang of
it now and remember to weigh
yourself daily, you don't have to
record unless you just want to but
use it to guage to where you are.

Breakfast

_____

_____

_____

_____

_____

_____

_____

_____

_____

Lunch

_____
_____
_____
_____
_____
_____
_____
_____

Supper

_____
_____
_____
_____
_____
_____

_____
_____
_____

Total Carbs

_____

Day Eleven

Breakfast

_____
_____
_____
_____
_____
_____
_____
_____
_____

Lunch

_____

_____

_____

_____

_____

_____

_____

_____

_____

Supper

_____

_____

_____

_____

_____

_____

_____

_____

_____

Total Carbs

_____

Day Twelve

Breakfast

_____
_____
_____
_____
_____
_____
_____
_____
_____

Lunch

_____

_____

_____

_____

_____

_____

_____

_____

_____

Supper

_____

_____

_____

_____

_____

_____

_____

_____

_____

Total Carbs

_____

Day Thirteen

Breakfast

_____
_____
_____
_____
_____
_____
_____
_____

Lunch

_____

_____

_____

_____

_____

_____

_____

_____

Supper

_____

_____

_____

_____

_____

_____

_____

_____

Total Carbs

_____

Day Fourteen

You should be showing at least a
one to three pound loss by now. If
not you need to double check that
you are not forgetting to write
down all the carbs you
eat-everything.

Breakfast

_____

_____

_____

_____

_____

_____

_____

_____

_____

Lunch

_____

_____

_____

_____

_____

_____

_____

_____

Supper

_____

_____

_____

_____

_____

_____

_____

_____

Total Carbs

_____

Day Fifteen

You need to a self evaluation at
this point and see how you are
doing. If you are not losing weight
try eating different foods. Don't be
afraid of any food, keep trying

until you find what is best for your body type.

Breakfast

_____

_____

_____

_____

_____

_____

_____

_____

_____

Lunch

_____

_____

_____

_____

_____

_____

_____

_____

_____

Supper

_____

_____

_____

_____

_____

_____

_____

_____

Total Carbs

_____

Day Sixteen

Breakfast

_____

_____

_____

_____

_____

_____

_____

_____

_____

Lunch

_____

_____

_____

_____

_____

_____

_____

_____

_____

Supper

_____

_____

_____

_____

_____

_____

_____

_____

_____

Total Carbs

_____

Day Seventeen

Breakfast

_____

_____

_____

_____

_____

_____

_____

_____

_____

Lunch

_____

————————————

————————————

————————————

————————————

————————————

————————————

————————————

————————————

Supper

————————————

————————————

————————————

————————————

————————————

————————————

————————————

————————————

————————————

Total Carbs

_____

Day Eighteen

Remember this is you plan and keep working on it and you will find as I have that you enjoy all the foods there are to be enjoyed if and that moderation in all things is the key to life and that you are truly the secret to all great success you can have in your life from permanent weight loss to anything you decide to do in life. Believe in yourself and keep your mout shut and your mind open and don't be negative toward yourself or anyone else and you will be happier and live longer.

Breakfast

_____

_____

_____

_____
_____
_____
_____

Lunch

_____
_____
_____
_____
_____
_____
_____

Supper

_____
_____
_____
_____
_____
_____
_____

Total Carbs

This booklet was written by me
Arthur Guess and I hope and pray
it has been of help to you.

If you would like to contact me
you can email me at
artguess@embarq.com